the

wellness

plan

belongs to:

....

For a Better Well-Designed World

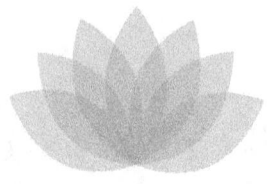

CREATE CHANGE. BE CHANGED.

Discover effective ways to be live a healthy lifestyle today.

Whether you're busy caregiving for loved ones, have no time for yourself, and have unsuccessfully tried so many diet/fitness/get-rich plans, here at ZenOmix Institute, you will learn how to design a wellness plan that works for you!

If you have any questions about the guide and join the newsletter, please email to info@zenomixinstitute.com.

Watch our video series on healthy habits.

Sign up for integrative health coaching.

Say "YES" to expressing your well-designed DNA.

Become a member of the ZenOmix Institute.

www.zenomixinstitute.com

the wellness plan

A GUIDE TO THE DNA OF
HEALTHY LIVING

WRITTEN BY DR. K. CHAN

Table of Contents

Part 3. The 7 Dimensions of Wellness

- Undated monthly planner
- Undated weekly planner
- The 7 dimensions of wellness
    1) Physical Wellness
    2) Intellectual Wellness
    3) Emotional Wellness
    4) Spiritual Wellness
    5) Social Wellness
    6) Occupational Wellness
    7) Environmental Wellness
- Celebrate your wellness plan
- Dating the well-designed me

Part 4. What's next?

References
Resources

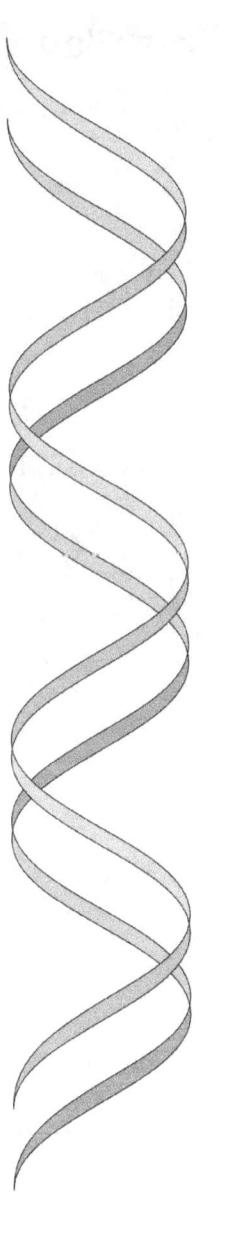

Part 1
What
is
the
wellness
plan?

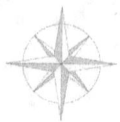

How to Use This Planner

What's Inside

- Seven Dimensions of Wellness:
  Core concepts of each dimensions
  (physical, intelligence, emotional, spiritual, social,
  occupational, environmental).
- List of Mini-Habit Tips.
- List of Mini-Changes Tips.
- Undated weekly planner sheets for SMARTER goals
  setting.
- Undated monthly planner sheets for SMARTER goals
  setting.
- Reflection questions to track your progress.
- Blank lined-pages for notes.

The Plan Layout

- Weekly intentions and goal setting prompts to track
  progress.
- Undated weekly plans from Sunday - Saturday section to
  set SMARTER goals for each dimension.
- Undated calendar to start and stop anytime.
- Specific reflective question per week to help uncover new
  ideas, core values, and dreams.
- Vision Page for creative visualization.

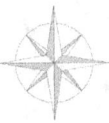

How to Succeed with Your Plan

1. Create your Vision Map: where do you see your 'well-designed self' at the end of 7-weeks, 6 months, 1 year, or 3 years.

2. Choose a strategy that works well with your DNA and environment to optimize your plan for wellness. Read more about the four strategies: gradual, chunking, laser-focused, or step-by-step in the wellness plan guide.

3. Define your mission statement to live a stress-free, healthy, compassionate life in a well-designed world.

4. Learn how different personality types can impact your plan, create, and maintain a wellness plan.

5. Stick with a systematic approach for self-evaluation. For example, you can reflect and journal in your guide at the end of the week, or check-in with an accountability buddy who will be also working on his/her wellness plan, or meet monthly with your health coach.

6. Be kind and compassionate toward yourself during this process of self-discovery.

7. Share your lessons learned and unlearned as you create your blueprint for a healthy well-designed you with family, friends and the world. Take a photo of your wellness plan, write a message or tweet an image of yourself on social media by tagging with #WellnessPlanDNA.

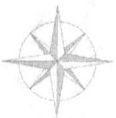

Introduction to the DNA of Healthy Living

At the beginning of each year, we often hear the different versions of the same type of New Year's resolutions:

- I want to exercise more.
- I want to be healthier.
- I want to lose weight
- I want to save more money.
- I want to be happy.

We buy into the latest trends for diet, weight loss, and exercise and stick with it for the first few weeks. We vowed to ourselves, to family and friends, and to the Higher God/Universe/Mother Nature that this year will be different. Studies still indicate that only 10% of the people who made New Year's resolutions are keeping their resolutions by the 6th month.

Given the array of solutions ranging from weight loss program, diet, calorie counting smartphone apps, budgeting tactics, and social media platforms, how is it possible that we are 'still' wishing for a healthier, happier life?

What's the real problem here?

Perhaps the real question is, 'Have we focused too much on the creating one-size fits all solutions here? Unexpected interruptions to a daily routine to eat sensibly, exercise, and sleep properly can derail your desire for getting healthy unless you can learn to expect barriers and adapt to a 'changing environment'.

Your Way. Your Style. *Your Plan*

A whole year passes by, and do you find yourself making the same list of resolutions (once again)?

The science of healthy living lies within you and the key to designing the best optimal wellness plan are based on your personality, environmental triggers and the seven dimensions of wellness. You are in control of your genetic potential for greatness, happiness, and optimal health.

You already know *'what'* you need to do.
This guide will teach you *'how to'* do it.

Live Your Best Well-Designed DNA

Your DNA (your blueprint) to healthy living is the product of the decisions, habits, and choices we make across seven dimensions:

(1) physical
(2) intellectual
(3) emotional
(4) social
(5) spiritual
(6) occupational
(7) environmental

Design the wellness plan based on your values and the dimension(s) in need of attention. Use this planner to reflect and journal any lessons learned and share your experiences with others. Feel free to post any new findings on the science of healthy living that resonated with you on social media with the hashtag #WellnessPlanDNA

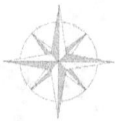

What happens if we neglect our wellness?

Science has shown that individuals who engaged mindfully about their health and wellness have a lower chance of developing the following diseases:

- Heart disease
- Obesity
- Diabetes
- Cancer
- Osteoporosis
- Alzheimer's Disease
- Lower Back Pain
- Chronic Fatigue
- Muscle Stiffness
- Moodiness, Depression, and Anxiety.
- Indigestion
- Gastrointestinal diseases
- Skin disorders (i.e. psoriasis, acnes)
- Cold/Flu
- Bacterial Infections

If we neglect our wellness, we increase our chances of developing these dis-eases (the absence of ease, peace, and energy for healthy living).

Capture your self-discovery and journey of transformation to a healthy blueprint of you.

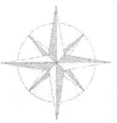

A SWOT Test
(strength, weakness, opportunity, & threat)

Self-evaluation is the first step toward developing personal accountability to making long-lasting changes and for developing a healthy genetic blueprint. Everyone has a different path to uncovering the DNA to healthy living because it is based on his/her genetics and non-genetic environmental factors. From that baseline, you will know the type of changes you want, what process will work for you, how much change you want to see, and when you want to see these incremental or substantial changes in creating your well-designed plan.

Let's do a SWOT test.
SWOT stands for Strengths, Weaknesses, Opportunities, and Threats.

Identify Your Own Strengths. Which dimension(s) do you gravitate to? Are you naturally strong in this dimension? Do you enjoy working in these area(s)?

Learn From Your Weaknesses. Which dimension(s) needs more attention? Do you have a strong desire to improve in this dimension but do not know how?

Find New Opportunities. Are there opportunities to make improvement or refinement in this dimension of wellness?

Be Mindful of Threats. Distractors, excuses, and obstacles can often derail our wellness plan. Can you identify possible threats so you can create new solutions or strategies to circumvent these barriers?

Mark "x" or "✓" in the dimension(s) boxes to indicate your strengths (S) & weakness (W) and possible opportunities (O) for improvement & threats (T) that distract you from healthy living.

Strength, Weakness, Opportunity, & Threats			
Dimension of Wellness	S	W	O T
Physical			
Intellectual			
Emotional			
Spiritual			
Social			
Occupational			
Environmental			
Total SWOT Findings			

You can focus more time on the dimension(s) with an indicator of W, O, and/or T while still engaging in the dimensions where your strengths (S) lie to help boost your confidence in creating a healthy life.

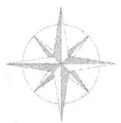

Wellness Vision Plan

Today:

Dimension of Wellness	My vision for myself in this dimension:
Physical	
Intellectual	
Emotional	
Spiritual	
Social	
Occupational	
Environmental	

Why is this overall wellness plan important to me now?

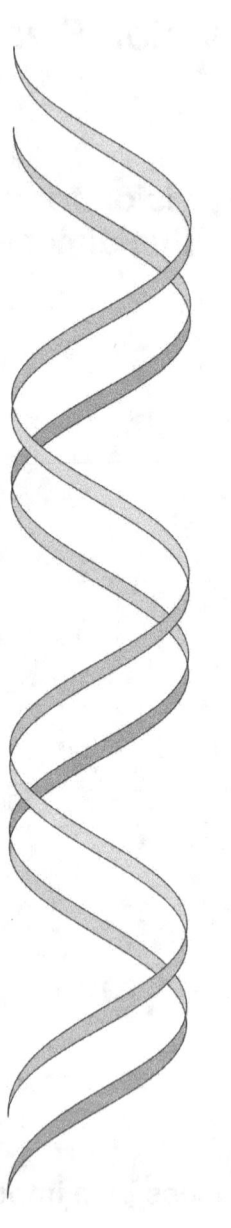

Part 2
Setting
up
the
wellness
plan

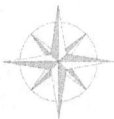

The SMARTER Method™

This planner journal is uniquely crafted to organize your dreams, goals, and purpose using The SMARTER Method™. You have the destination in mind, but there is no map, no direction, and simply no end in sight. Using this planner and journal, you can design your roadmap using the undated monthly calendar, weekly planner, and reflective pages.

Carve your path with The SMARTER Method™. You can start your weekly plan anytime during the year. The weekly schedule is undated so that you can start in January or March. You can track a 3-month plan, take a break and repeat. You can make a weekly planner for your work life and a separate one for your personal life. Make your plan work for you!

The SMARTER Method™ stands for:

- ❏ Specificity
- ❏ Measurable
- ❏ Achievable
- ❏ Realistic
- ❏ Timed
- ❏ Enthusiasm
- ❏ Reason

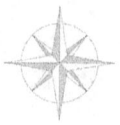

SPECIFICITY

Make your goal specific, personal, and meaningful. When adding 'specificity' to your goal, ask yourself: What aspect(s) of this goal am I trying to achieve?

Here is a typical goal:

"I want to <u>lose weight</u> this year."

Rewrite the goal using The SMARTER Method™ :

"I want to <u>lose the 10 pounds that I gained from last year</u>."

Notice the underlined parts of the sentence to highlight the different components of The SMARTER Method™.

Why is the goal SMARTER?

Add specificity to the 'task' you are trying to achieve. How much weight loss is reasonable? If 10 pounds was gained in a year, it seems possible to lose the 10 pounds within a year. If you want to live a healthy lifestyle, which aspects of your current routine are you willing to change ? Can you maintain this new habit? Start with a small goal. Small wins will build confidence, leading to Big Wins.

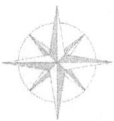

MEASURABLE

Define a way to measure your goals. Make goals measurable by asking yourself: by how much or how many? Measure your task to completion in terms of value, expectations, and importance. Keep in mind that measurement is usually represented in units (i.e. per day, per month, # of ... etc.)

Here is a typical goal:

"I want to <u>lose weight</u> this year."

Rewrite the goal using The SMARTER Method™ :

"I want to lose the <u>10 pounds I gained from last year</u> by substituting <u>one meal per day</u> with a vegetarian meal . . . "

Notice the underlined parts of the sentence to highlight the different components of The SMARTER Method™.

Why is the goal SMARTER?

The goal is to lose weight and the task is to change an "eating habit." Making small incremental changes in your routine helps you transform a new change into a new habit. Over time, the new habit becomes a part of your natural behavior. Changing one meal per day is measurable. You either had or didn't have a vegetarian meal per day.

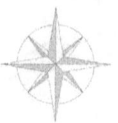

ACHIEVABLE

Don't put yourself up for failure by making goals unachievable and unattainable. Conduct a SWOT (strength, weakness, opportunity, and threat) self-analysis. Know your strengths and weaknesses in making new changes in different stages of your life. Does the timing make sense now? Be honest. If you need help, ask for help. If you need to postpone this task where you have time and energy, do so.

Here is a typical goal:

"I want to <u>lose weight </u>this year."

Rewrite the goal using The SMARTER Method™ :

"I want to lose the <u>10 pounds I gained from last year</u> by substituting <u>one meal per day </u>with a vegetarian meal with <u>my friend, Sarah (who is a vegetarian)</u> . . . "

Why is the goal SMARTER?

With a more specific and measurable goal, you can incorporate 'external triggers or cues' to help you achieve and attain your goal. Adding one vegetarian meal to your new eating habit will take a time to adjust. Use this opportunity to gain support from someone who is already doing this task.

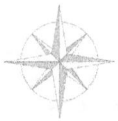

REALISTIC

Complete goals with action based on your values, reasonable expectations, and accountability. Clarify the steps to reaching your goal. Ask yourself: Am I asking a reasonable amount of time, energy, and support to work on this goal?

Here is a typical goal:

"I want to <u>lose weight</u> this year."

Rewrite the goal using The SMARTER Method™:

I want to lose the <u>10 pounds I gained from last year</u> by substituting <u>one meal per day</u> with a vegetarian meal with <u>my friend, Sarah (who is a vegetarian)</u> during my <u>work lunch hour</u>. . . "

Why is the goal SMARTER?

Realistically achieve your goals within the constraints of time and space. Having a vegetarian meal during lunch time with a friend who is a vegetarian will help you develop the new habit since adding the vegetarian meal option during dinner with family and friends may be influenced by others' food preferences.

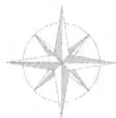

TIMED

Add a deadline or a timeframe to work on the goal. This helps you to plan accordingly. We often underestimate the time to get things done. Multiply the amount of time you think it will take to complete a task by a factor of 2. This will give you room and space to adapt to the new habit and adjust for any delays.

Here is a typical goal:

"I want to <u>lose weight </u>this year."

Rewrite the goal using The SMARTER Method™ :

"I want to lose the <u>10 pounds I gained from last year</u> by substituting <u>one meal per day </u>with a vegetarian meal with <u>my friend, Sarah (who is a vegetarian</u>) during my <u>work lunch hour</u> for the <u>next 4 weeks</u> . . . "

Why is the goal SMARTER?

Making new habit(s) as a part of your lifestyle will take some time. Establishing deadlines and timeframe for time and space allows you to reflect on the achievements made and any obstacles encountered. If you were not able to achieve the task by the deadline, adjust the time. This information also helps you to know your rate and pace of completing a task and goal. If the time frame or deadline has been achieved, it is time to reward yourself!

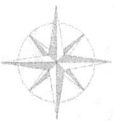

ENTHUSIASM

If you are excited about your goal, the end product, and reward, you will have the physical and mental energy to work toward your goal, even when the going get tough. You will have the motivation and determination to break the wall to any obstacles, jump over any speedbumps, and defend yourself against any curve balls thrown at you.

Here is a typical goal:

"I want to <u>lose weight</u> this year."

Rewrite the goal using The SMARTER Method™ :

"I want to lose the <u>10 pounds I gained from last year</u> by substituting <u>one meal per day</u> with a vegetarian meal with <u>my friend, Sarah (who is a vegetarian)</u> during my <u>work lunch hour</u> for <u>next 4 weeks</u> because <u>I am excited to feel better</u> . . . "

Why is the goal SMARTER?

Excitement about achieving the goal is needed to transform the new change into a new habit. Adding internal and external rewards in finishing the task can also give you a boost of confidence. When you are about to give up and revert to your old habit, revisit this feeling of happiness about achieving your goals.

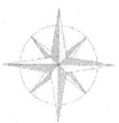

REASON

Sometimes we have strong desires to achieve a goal, but without a clear reason, it can be challenging to hold yourself (or others) accountable to achieving this goal, especially during challenging times. You will be dedicated to completing your goal with a meaningful and personal reason.

Here is a typical goal:

"I want to <u>lose weight</u> this year."

Rewrite the goal using The SMARTER Method™ :

"I want to lose the <u>10 pounds I gained from last year</u> by substituting <u>one meal per day</u> with a vegetarian meal with <u>my friend, Sarah (who is a vegetarian)</u> during my <u>work lunch hour</u> for the <u>next 4 weeks</u> because <u>I am excited to feel better about my physical, mental and emotional well-being</u>."

Why is the goal SMARTER?

There are many good reasons to live a happy and happy life. Make your reason personal and right for you. In this example, changing the eating habit will help with weight management, which may result in having more energy to spend with family and friends.

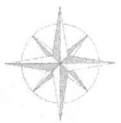

Your Best Year Yet with
The SMARTER Method™

The wellness plan includes well-designed words with undated pages. Space is provided for you to start on any one wellness dimension anytime and anywhere.

Using The SMARTER Method™ to set your wellness goals for each dimension.

Use this checklist to define SMARTER Goals:

- ☐ Specificity
- ☐ Measurable
- ☐ Achievable
- ☐ Realistic
- ☐ Timed
- ☐ Enthusiasm
- ☐ Reason

At the end of each week, there is a series of reflective questions to help capture what you learned and unlearned in each dimension.

Use The SMARTER Method™ to plan for optimal wellness for your well-designed lifestyle.

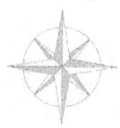

Your Strategy to Optimal Wellness

Pick 1 of the 4 approaches based on your time-commitment:
gradual, chunking, laser-focused, or step-by-step.

☐ **Gradual Approach**, where you will focus on only *one wellness dimension every 7-weeks* over the course of a year. For example, Physical Wellness from Week 1 - Week 7; Intellectual Wellness from Week 8 - Week 14 ... etc.
(a 7-weekly plan for each dimension).

☐ **Chunking Approach**, where you will focus on *one wellness dimension per month.* For example, Physical wellness for the 1st month (Jan), Intellectual Wellness for the 2nd month (Feb) ... etc. (a monthly/4-week plan).

☐ **Laser-Focused Approach**, where you will focus on *one wellness dimension per week* over the next seven weeks. For example, Intellectual wellness for Week 1; Physical Wellness for Week 2 ... etc. (a variable weekly plan).

☐ **Step-by-Step Approach**, where you will work on *one wellness dimension per day,* thus covering all seven dimensions of wellness every week.
(a daily plan).

Longer Time Commitment

Shorter & Intense Time Commitment

Mix & Match the Plan.
Try each style and see what works best for you.

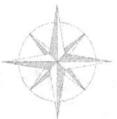

Mini-Habits of Wellness

Developing new habits to foster life-long changes may sound like a daunting task and will take some time, resources, and commitment. Sometimes, the fear of failure or the lack of follow-through impedes us from even taking the first step toward action.

Thus, the wellness plan will help you develop "mini-habits of wellness" where we will focus on making incremental changes during micro-moments throughout the day. For example, the brief transient time spent waiting in traffic (i.e. micro-moment) can be used to practice deep breathing (mini-habit).

Over time, these mini-habits will become a part of your routine, schedule, and lifestyle, which at that time you would no longer need to think, analyze and negotiate the time and benefits. Your brain will act and react naturally. By then, your body, mind, and heart are connected to your new DNA of healthy living!

Using the wellness plan to uncover the 7 dimensions of wellness, you will learn to

- overcome impulsive urges to break your new mini-habit.
- focus on creating balance and harmony.
- develop environmental triggers to foster positive changes.
- increase your energy for a well-designed life.
- discover the strategy that works and doesn't work based on your own terms.

Mini Changes Ideas
Add one (or more) of these ideas in your wellness plan.

- Drink a glass of warm water in the morning.
- Substitute a cup of coffee with a cup of herbal tea.
- Add fruits to your meals.
- Walk for 10 minutes before you get to work.
- Walk around the block before you get to work.
- Take the stairs at work or at home.
- Take a 15 minutes walk during your afternoon break.
- Plan a lunch date with a colleague or friend you haven't seen for awhile.
- Reduce your intake of salt by 25% this week.
- Eat fish at least once a week.
- Park your car far away to get into the habit of walking.
- Add dried fruits to your salads.
- Instead of cookies and chips, snack on 10 almonds or nuts.
- Add a 10 minute walk at least three times a week.
- Enjoy 2 oz. of dark chocolate after your meal.
- Add one more servings of vegetables to your meal.
- Try new vegetables once a month.
- Instead of whip cream, add some fresh berries on desserts.
- Do at least one push-up per day.
- Do at least 25 jumping stacks or jump per week.
- Schedule your dentist appointment.
- Drink a glass of warm water before each meal.
- Drink a glass of hot tea after each meal.
- Add 10 minutes of resistance strength training to your exercises.
- Learn a new word each week.
- Add calcium supplements to your diet.
- Cook with olive oil or coconut oil.
- Treat yourself to a massage this week.
- Drink peppermint tea after a meal to help with digestion.
- Reduce your intake of sugar by 25% this week.

Some More Mini Changes Ideas

Add one (or more) of these ideas in your wellness plan.

- Try a new recipe from a different region from where you are living.
- Switch from white bread to wheat, whole grained bread.
- Reduce your television and movie watching by 25%.
- Add Vitamin C to your diet.
- Get some sun exposure for 10 minutes (max) to activate your Vitamin D level.
- Volunteer in your community or online for public service at least once a month.
- Find time for Pilates exercise for 30 minutes per week.
- Bring flowers or plants to your workplace.
- Surprise your co-workers by treating them an extra cup of coffee or tea.
- Eat breakfast.
- Reduce your intake of caffeine by 25%.
- Spend time with Nature at least one weekend per month.
- Draw or doodle for 15 minutes in the morning.
- Find time for yoga for 30 minutes at least 3 times per week.
- Get to know your neighbor.
- Learn a new name this week.
- Treat someone for free lunch this week.
- Learn to budget and live below your means.
- Pick up a newspaper and read an article.
- Recycle papers or cans this week.
- Write a 'thank you' card to an old friend or mentor.
- Turn off your mobile phone for a weekend this month.
- Live wirelessly for one weekend this month.
- Read a book from a new author.
- Attend a book discussion at your local library.
- Recite a mantra during your meditation.
- Reduce your internet shopping by 25%.
- Add lavender oil to your bath.
- Meditate at least for one minute each morning.

This Year I will

_____

_____

_____

_____

_____

_____

_____

Monthly SMARTER Goal Setting
YEAR _____

I will focus on

_____

wellness this month.

My SMARTER Goals are:

I will focus on

_____

wellness this month.

My SMARTER Goals are:

I will focus on

_____

wellness this month.

My SMARTER Goals are:

I will focus on

_____

wellness this month

My SMARTER Goals are:

I will focus on

_____

wellness this month.

My SMARTER Goals are:

I will focus on

_____

wellness this month.

My SMARTER Goals are:

My Six-Month Vision and Goals

_____

_____

_____

_____

Monthly SMARTER Goal Setting
YEAR _____

JULY

I will focus on

_____

wellness this month.

My SMARTER Goals are:

AUGUST

I will focus on

_____

wellness this month.

My SMARTER Goals are:

SEPTEMBER

I will focus on

_____

wellness this month.

My SMARTER Goals are:

OCTOBER

I will focus on

_____

wellness this month.

My SMARTER Goals are:

NOVEMBER

I will focus on

_____

wellness this month.

My SMARTER Goals are:

DECEMBER

I will focus on

_____

wellness this month.

My SMARTER Goals are:

My Six-Month Vision and Goals

_____

_____

_____

_____

Monthly SMARTER Goal Setting
YEAR _____

JANUARY

I will focus on

_____

wellness this month.

My SMARTER Goals are:

FEBRUARY

I will focus on

_____

wellness this month.

My SMARTER Goals are:

MARCH

I will focus on

_____

wellness this month.

My SMARTER Goals are:

APRIL

I will focus on

_____

wellness this month.

My SMARTER Goals are:

MAY

I will focus on

_____

wellness this month.

My SMARTER Goals are:

JUNE

I will focus on

_____

wellness this month.

My SMARTER Goals are:

My Six-Month Vision and Goals

_____

_____

_____

_____

Monthly SMARTER Goal Setting
YEAR _____

JULY

I will focus on

_____

wellness this month.

My SMARTER Goals are:

AUGUST

I will focus on

_____

wellness this month.

My SMARTER Goals are:

SEPTEMBER

I will focus on

_____

wellness this month.

My SMARTER Goals are:

OCTOBER

I will focus on

_____

wellness this month.

My SMARTER Goals are:

NOVEMBER

I will focus on

_____

wellness this month.

My SMARTER Goals are:

DECEMBER

I will focus on

_____

wellness this month.

My SMARTER Goals are:

My Six-Month Vision and Goals

_____

_____

_____

_____

I will see my self-directed
transformation using
the wellness plan by

_____

(date)

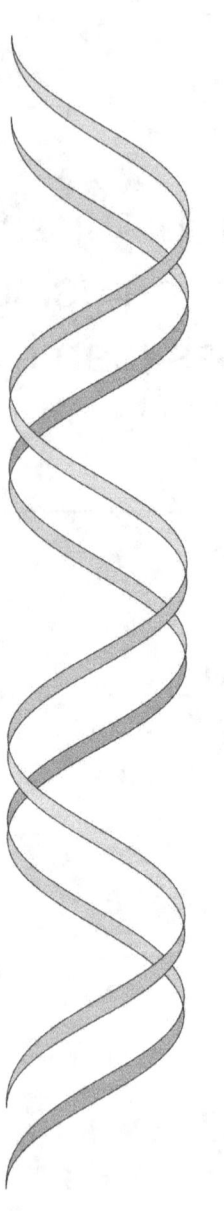

Part 3
The 7
Dimensions
of
Wellness

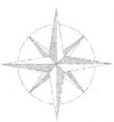

Physical Wellness

Physical Wellness is the sense of feeling connected with your body to move smoothly, gracefully, and functionally. Working on your physical wellness will not only help you move better, but also feel better (emotional wellness), think better (intellectual wellness), serve better (spiritual wellness), connect better (social wellness), work better (occupational wellness), and create a better world to live in (environmental wellness).

As we age, our physical wellness will evolve accordingly in different stages of our lives. In your earlier years, you want to have the energy to move freely, travel, and jumpstart your life purpose. In your later stages of life, you want to have the energy to move gracefully, be there for your growing children, see your grandchildren, or still maintain a sense of independence. When we train our muscle well with exercises, mindful movements, and a positive attitude, our body can store these mind-body connection memories and help us move gracefully throughout our life span.

At any point in time, unexpected life situations may challenge your physical health: you've gotten ill, you're taking care of your loved ones, or you're going through a rough patch at work. How does your body function when your energy level is suboptimal?

It is important that you have a clear basic understanding of your physical conditions so you know when to accelerate, slow down or even shift to a neutral gear to cruise through this moment in time.

When does physical wellness matter?

The life-course perspective gives us a window to understanding how and when physical wellness matters. Today's experiences and exposures can influence tomorrow's health like a timeline. Health trajectories are particular effective during critical and sensitive period (when and how long you engage in physical activity). The timing of events and exposure to external factors can have an impact on the manifestation of disease and well-being.

How does the physical wellness impact our body in cellular level?

Exercise is linked to methylation of a specific gene which results in a chemical structural change in the DNA. This change, known as epigenetic, can increase or decrease the risk for chronic diseases. Methylation of pro-inflammatory genes can turn off the biological pathway that would have increase the risk for chronic diseases such as heart disease, cancer, and obesity.

Aging process is linked to the length of telomeres, which are specific end-region of the DNA strand and their roles are involved with protecting the DNA from damage during cell division and replication. As we age, our telomeres shorten naturally. Interestingly, an individual with a sedentary lifestyle has shorter telomeres compared to someone who exercises regularly. Thus, exercise may have the power to slow down the aging process.

The wellness plan for physical wellness

Exercises improve the strength and endurance of the heart condition and the cardiac output, which measures how much blood the heart can pump. Thus, exercise can help increase the heart efficiency to pump blood and decrease the work load the heart has to perform at any level of activity (walking, running, and stress under work).

Guidelines for Exercises

1) **Intensity of the exercise** focuses on a target heart rate or at a level of exercise intensity. Modify the speed and incline setting for a treadmill exercise.

2) **Duration of training** is the time frame designated for the physical activity. For beginners, start within a range between 20-30 minutes of exercise and include a 5-10 minute warming up before and after exercise. For relaxation, end your exercise with a meditation.

3) **Frequency of training** is usually expressed in the number of sessions per week. At minimum, training programs should be done 3-5 times a week.

4) **Specificity (type of exercise)** refers to the performance of activities in training. Not all exercise has the identical physiological benefits. If you are using swimming for aerobic training, the benefits from swimming aren't the same as running and vice versa.

Add walking, running, stair climbing, cycling, cross country skiing, long distance swimming, and other activity that increase the heart rate throughout your wellness plan.

MY NOTES

MY NOTES

MY NOTES

MY NOTES

MY NOTES

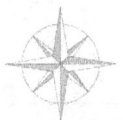

Vision Page for
Physical Wellness

MONTH:

Wellness	
WEEK # 1	**SMARTER Weekly Goals**
SUN	
MON	
TUES	
WED	
THURS	
FRI	
SAT	

Week # 1
Reflective Responses:

If time was not an issue, how much more time would I dedicate myself to physical activity per week, and can I make one small incremental change toward fulfilling this wellness goal this week?

_____

_____

_____

_____

_____

_____

_____

_____

_____

_____

_____

_____

_____

_____

_____

_____

_____

_____

_____

_____

_____

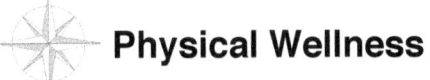 **Physical Wellness**

MONTH:

Wellness	
WEEK # 2	**SMARTER Weekly Goals**
SUN	
MON	
TUES	
WED	
THURS	
FRI	
SAT	

Week # 2
Reflective Responses:

What types of physical activity bring me joy when I was a
child and can I make one small incremental change
toward fulfilling this wellness goal this week?

_____

_____

_____

_____

_____

_____

_____

_____

_____

_____

_____

_____

_____

_____

_____

_____

_____

_____

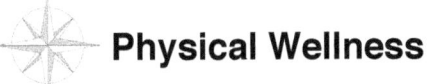 **Physical Wellness**

MONTH:

Wellness	
WEEK # 3	**SMARTER Weekly Goals**
SUN	
MON	
TUES	
WED	
THURS	
FRI	
SAT	

Week # 3
Reflective Responses:
What physical activities do I enjoy alone or with friends?
Can I make one small incremental change toward
fulfilling this wellness goal?

_____

_____

_____

_____

_____

_____

_____

_____

_____

_____

_____

_____

_____

_____

_____

_____

_____

_____

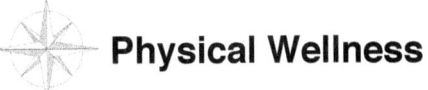 **Physical Wellness**

MONTH:

Wellness	
WEEK # 4	**SMARTER Weekly Goals**
SUN	
MON	
TUES	
WED	
THURS	
FRI	
SAT	

Week # 4
Reflective Responses:

How is my body feeling usually before and after a workout? Do I have physical or mental fatigue (or both)? If I am tired before my workout, can I make one small incremental change toward fulfilling this wellness goal? (i.e. mental preparation, better diet, more sleep ... etc)

_____

_____

_____

_____

_____

_____

_____

_____

_____

_____

_____

_____

_____

_____

_____

_____

_____

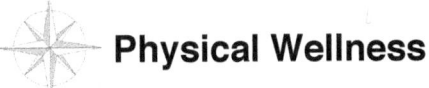 **Physical Wellness**

MONTH:

Wellness	
WEEK # 5	**SMARTER Weekly Goals**
SUN	
MON	
TUES	
WED	
THURS	
FRI	
SAT	

Week # 5
Reflective Responses:

What types of food am I eating before and after the workout? If my goal is to lose weight, build muscle, increase flexibility, or increase strength, can I make one small incremental change toward fulfilling this goal?

_____

_____

_____

_____

_____

_____

_____

_____

_____

_____

_____

_____

_____

_____

_____

_____

_____

_____

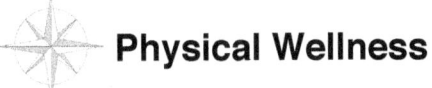 **Physical Wellness**

MONTH:

Wellness	
WEEK # 6	**SMARTER Weekly Goals**
SUN	
MON	
TUES	
WED	
THURS	
FRI	
SAT	

Week # 6
Reflective Responses:

What is my routine and process that I use to prepare for a workout (i.e. planning the time to workout, getting gym bag ready, or call up a friend to work out)?

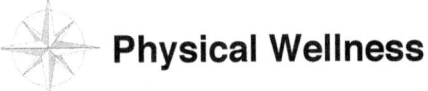 **Physical Wellness**

MONTH:

Wellness	
WEEK # 7	**SMARTER Weekly Goals**
SUN	
MON	
TUES	
WED	
THURS	
FRI	
SAT	

Week # 7
Reflective Responses:

What are some reasons (or excuses) that I have told myself that "it is okay to skip a workout"? (i.e. I am not in the mood, I can't find my lucky shoes ... etc)

_____

_____

_____

_____

_____

_____

_____

_____

_____

_____

_____

_____

_____

_____

_____

_____

_____

_____

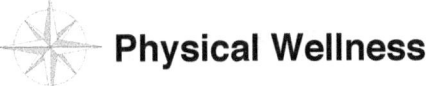 **Physical Wellness**

WELLNESS REFLECTIONS:

What brought you positive energy from this dimension of wellness? What were your hopes, inspirations, and dreams during this new change?

What brought you negative energy from this dimension of wellness? Did you experience any obstacles, distractions, or guilty feeling toward new change?

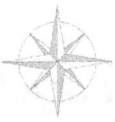

Intellectual Wellness

Intellectual wellness is how well we stay challenged and curious about things in life. Explore new hobbies with your creativity. Learn new skills. Read new subjects. Challenge your mind by playing the devil advocate. Throughout the day, our mind is constantly making decisions, and we have two brains to help us make choices.

To function effectively under different conditions, Mother Nature developed a two-part decision-making process: **Fast brain system 1 and Slow brain system.**

Because there are so many different external environmental factors grabbing our attention and pulling us in multiple directions, we need to make it easier for our brain to decide, take action (or not) and think fast and slow.

Fast brain system 1 helps you make a decision that requires little thinking and needs only few set of tasks and skills that use minimal resources and fuel. Think of the task of brushing your teeth after you wake up. You don't spend time negotiating in your mind whether it is a good idea or not. This task is automatic, comes naturally to you, and most importantly, requires little brain power to act.

Slow brain system 2 helps you think through a problem, analyze the situation, and make choices among different options. For example, the decision to buy a new house requires thoughtful consideration of various factors: house preferences, affordability, neighborhood, school system, transportation from home to work. This task requires brain power to think critically, analyze and to interrupt the data presented to you.

Ways to Enhance Intellectual Power

- Exercise
- Meditation
- Hand-on Experience

Exercise helps increase cognitive function and creative thinking by providing the 'energy food' needed for the brain cells to function properly and to transmit signal to make connection between nerve cells to act and react appropriately. Simple task (or old habit) would require less connection and less energy, and thus, more complex task (such as developing a new habit) that required either physical expenditure of energy, strength, or mental capacity to analyze and criticize will take up more connections, and thus need more energy

Meditation is the second way to increase brain power. You can start with focusing your attention on the flame of a candle, the petal of a flower, the breath sensation through your nose, or even close your eyes and focus on the space between the brows. The practice of meditation will increase your sense of empathy, compassion, and clarity for oneself and others. When the mind connects to your higher purpose in a clutter-free space, your brain will have the mental energy to innovate and create new ideas.

Hand-on experience can help develop and refine motor skills which requires brain power to coordinate appropriate, specific physical and mental movements. Problem solving activity, creating crafts, and gardening are examples that involve detailed coordination. When you learn a new musical instrument, cooking a new recipe, or driving to a new place, these activities will also increase your brain power.

MY NOTES

MY NOTES

MY NOTES

MY NOTES

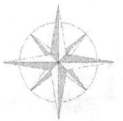

Vision Page for
Intellectual Wellness

MONTH:

Wellness	
WEEK # 1	**SMARTER Weekly Goals**
SUN	
MON	
TUES	
WED	
THURS	
FRI	
SAT	

Week # 1
Reflective Responses:

List the skills that people often ask for your help. If time was not an issue, what new skills would you like to learn? What is stopping you? Can you get some hand-on experience by shadowing someone, working on a team project, and enrolling in an online course?

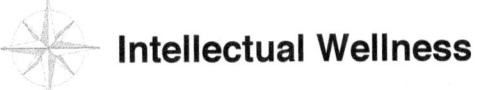 **Intellectual Wellness**

MONTH:

Wellness	
WEEK # 2	**SMARTER Weekly Goals**
SUN	
MON	
TUES	
WED	
THURS	
FRI	
SAT	

Week # 2
Reflective Responses:

The Fast Brain system 1 dominates the Slow Brain system 2. Can you create environmental cues to trick your slow brain system 2 to act like the fast brain system 1? (i.e. putting your running shoes and gym bag next to your workbag)

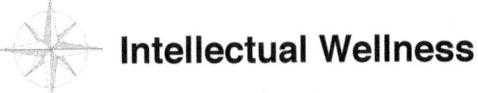 **Intellectual Wellness**

MONTH:

Wellness	
WEEK # 3	**SMARTER Weekly Goals**
SUN	
MON	
TUES	
WED	
THURS	
FRI	
SAT	

Week # 3
Reflective Responses:

List your achievements, awards, and honors. Are you using these skills or knowledge in your creative work or at home? If not, are there ways you can combine your achievements into your current work?

_____

_____

_____

_____

_____

_____

_____

_____

_____

_____

_____

_____

_____

_____

_____

_____

_____

_____

_____

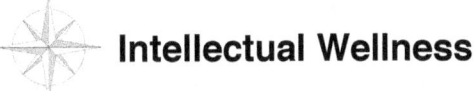 **Intellectual Wellness**

MONTH:

Wellness	
WEEK # 4	**SMARTER Weekly Goals**
SUN	
MON	
TUES	
WED	
THURS	
FRI	
SAT	

Week # 4
Reflective Responses:

List the books that made you think critically, change your mind on a subject, connected with you emotionally.

_____

_____

_____

_____

_____

_____

_____

_____

_____

_____

_____

_____

_____

_____

_____

_____

_____

_____

_____

_____

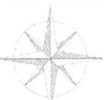 **Intellectual Wellness**

MONTH:

Wellness	
WEEK # 5	**SMARTER Weekly Goals**
SUN	
MON	
TUES	
WED	
THURS	
FRI	
SAT	

Week # 5
Reflective Responses:

List any new educational subjects (or courses) you would take now, if money or time was not an issue. Can you read a book or blog on this subject, take an online course, or even shadow someone who is teaching the subject.

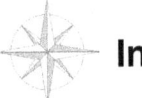 **Intellectual Wellness**

MONTH:

Wellness	
WEEK # 6	**SMARTER Weekly Goals**
SUN	
MON	
TUES	
WED	
THURS	
FRI	
SAT	

Week # 6
Reflective Responses:

Set your timer and meditate for two minutes. It is important to declutter your mind so random thoughts are not distracting you during your meditation. Write down your thoughts, worries, or concerns before you begin your meditation. After your meditation, share any new ideas or revelations after the meditation practice.

_____

_____

_____

_____

_____

_____

_____

_____

_____

_____

_____

_____

_____

_____

_____

_____

_____

_____

_____

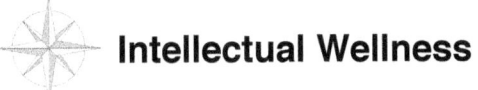 **Intellectual Wellness**

MONTH:

Wellness	
WEEK # 7	**SMARTER Weekly Goals**
SUN	
MON	
TUES	
WED	
THURS	
FRI	
SAT	

Week # 7
Reflective Responses:

Exercise can help boost brain power. Try to listen to an audiobook while you are running or indoor cycling. Write down how your mind and body feels after your workout. What types of mini-exercise can you add to your day to increase your brain power?

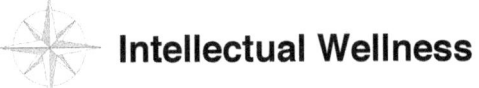 **Intellectual Wellness**

WELLNESS REFLECTIONS:

What brought you positive energy from this dimension of wellness? What were your hopes, inspirations, and dreams during this new change?

What brought you negative energy from this dimension of wellness? Did you experience any obstacles, distractions, or guilty feeling toward new change?

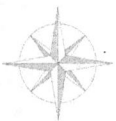

Emotional Wellness

Emotional wellness is how well we are connected with our values, beliefs, and feelings about ourselves, our experiences, and our interaction between ourselves and the experience. Emotions can impact our genetic expression and vice versa; our genetic expression can have an influence on our emotions. We have emotions based on our reaction to experiences, as well as emotions that were imprinted into our genome passed down from our ancestry.

Reflective writing is a great way to uncover these hidden emotions. Emotional wellness is a personalized journey for oneself. Appreciate yourself. Find balance and purpose in what you are doing, at work, at home, or in your hobbies.

Emotional wellness involves understanding yourself and others. It takes a little work to dive inside and into others. Connect with others wholeheartedly.

The four pillars of emotional intelligence that impact our overall emotional wellness are:

- Self-Awareness
- Self-Management
- Social Awareness
- Social Management

Four Pillars of Emotional Wellness

	Self	Social
Awareness	Emotional Stability Self-Esteem Self-Identify Personal Leadership	Compassion Empathy Connection Public Service Observational Mindfulness
Management	Self-Control Self-Worth Resilience Stress-Management Reflective	Appreciation Team Building Collective Impact Communication Adaptive Flexibility

Attributes and examples of four pillars of emotional wellness.

MY NOTES

MY NOTES

MY NOTES

MY NOTES

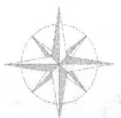

Vision Page for
Emotional Wellness

MONTH:

Wellness	
WEEK # 1	**SMARTER Weekly Goals**
SUN	
MON	
TUES	
WED	
THURS	
FRI	
SAT	

Week # 1
Reflective Responses:

List the most beautiful moments in your life. Describe these memories using your five senses (the scent, sound, taste, touch, and sight of the memory). Can you find or recognize these similar characteristics in the present moment.

_____

_____

_____

_____

_____

_____

_____

_____

_____

_____

_____

_____

_____

_____

_____

_____

_____

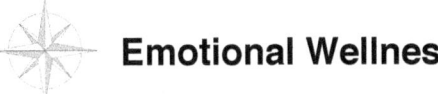 **Emotional Wellness**

MONTH:

Wellness	
WEEK # 2	**SMARTER Weekly Goals**
SUN	
MON	
TUES	
WED	
THURS	
FRI	
SAT	

Week # 2
Reflective Responses:

List the process that you use to declutter your closet.
Take a honest look at the stuff and what would your stuff
say about you? Are you holding onto anything that brings
your discomfort, sadness and hurt? Why are still holding
onto this?

_____

_____

_____

_____

_____

_____

_____

_____

_____

_____

_____

_____

_____

_____

_____

_____

_____

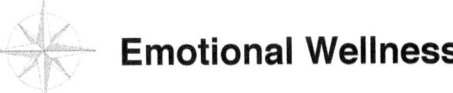 **Emotional Wellness**

MONTH:

Wellness	
WEEK # 3	**SMARTER Weekly Goals**
SUN	
MON	
TUES	
WED	
THURS	
FRI	
SAT	

Week # 3
Reflective Responses:

List food that you go to when you are feeling sad. Why does this food bring comfort to you? List ways to find a healthier type of comfort here.

_____

_____

_____

_____

_____

_____

_____

_____

_____

_____

_____

_____

_____

_____

_____

_____

_____

_____

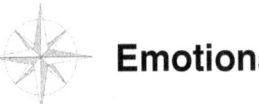 **Emotional Wellness**

MONTH:

Wellness	
WEEK # 4	**SMARTER Weekly Goals**
SUN	
MON	
TUES	
WED	
THURS	
FRI	
SAT	

Week # 4
Reflective Responses:

If your salary was cut in half, list the essential things you would spend money on. What are the new "Must Haves" and new "Wants/Desires". Do you notice any items that you are currently overspending on? Is there an emotional attachment that is difficult to let go? Why?

_____

_____

_____

_____

_____

_____

_____

_____

_____

_____

_____

_____

_____

_____

_____

_____

_____

_____

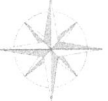 **Emotional Wellness**

MONTH:

Wellness	
WEEK # 5	**SMARTER Weekly Goals**
SUN	
MON	
TUES	
WED	
THURS	
FRI	
SAT	

Week # 5
Reflective Responses:

List the people who make you feel empowered. The attributes which you see in others are exhibited in you as well. How can you empower others in similar ways?

_____

_____

_____

_____

_____

_____

_____

_____

_____

_____

_____

_____

_____

_____

_____

_____

_____

_____

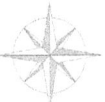 **Emotional Wellness**

MONTH:

Wellness	
WEEK # 6	**SMARTER Weekly Goals**
SUN	
MON	
TUES	
WED	
THURS	
FRI	
SAT	

Week # 6
Reflective Responses:
List the ways you can make a friend laugh when he/she is feeling sad. When you are too hard on yourself, give yourself the same pep talk and laugh like no one is watching.

_____

_____

_____

_____

_____

_____

_____

_____

_____

_____

_____

_____

_____

_____

_____

_____

_____

_____

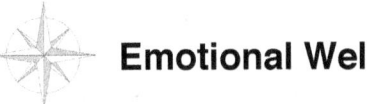 **Emotional Wellness**

MONTH:

Wellness	
WEEK # 7	**SMARTER Weekly Goals**
SUN	
MON	
TUES	
WED	
THURS	
FRI	
SAT	

Week # 7
Reflective Responses:

List the people who have been critical, judgmental, and mean to you (and is one of the people you?). Look at this list and sprinkle seeds of grace and compassion to them. Forgive them and let go of them.

_____

_____

_____

_____

_____

_____

_____

_____

_____

_____

_____

_____

_____

_____

_____

_____

_____

_____

_____

_____

_____

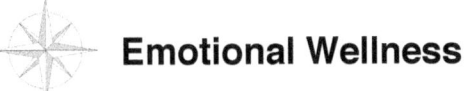 **Emotional Wellness**

WELLNESS REFLECTIONS:

What brought you positive energy from this dimension of wellness? What were your hopes, inspirations, and dreams during this new change?

What brought you negative energy from this dimension of wellness? Did you experience any obstacles, distractions, or guilty feeling toward new change?

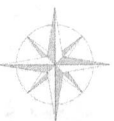

Spiritual Wellness

Spiritual wellness is how well you have a strong understanding of your purpose in life, how to experience love, joy, and peace, and even sadness. By understanding our spiritual wellness, it can help ourselves and others to achieve happiness and peace as a society as a human spirit.

We all have a sense of empathy, and we want to connect with others. But sometimes the busyness of life, we forget we are a part of a larger community of well-beings.

Spiritual wellness can be channeled through a personalized center meditative awareness. Deep breathing is a gift that you can tap into.

How do we engage in active breathing?

Deep breathing can train the body's reaction to a stressful situation to function gracefully. It calms the mind and reduces the production of stress hormone. When we are stressed, we tend to breathe through the chest, and this type of rapid breathing is unhealthy to our health over time.

Allow the breath to draw you into the space of stillness. Use this space of stillness to be present. This is the place of perfect peace. Continue to stay centered in the stillness for a few more minutes. Let thoughts enter your mind. Acknowledge them, be with them, see them as for what they are, thoughts. With clarity and space, visualize your mission, purpose, and the change your heart desires. Carry this mental imagery in your heart, and use the power of intention to awaken your energy to create a footprint of joy, happiness, and peace in this world.

Meditation 101

1. Find a comfortable position either sitting on the floor, chair, or lying down.

2. Gently close your eyes and focus your attention on your breath. Feel how your breath moves in and out of your nose.

3. Focus on your breath using all our five senses. Relax and deepen your peaceful body through the breath. Inhale through the nose and exhale through the mouth.

4. Release any tension you may be holding with each exhalation. Exhale with a thought of 'joy, peace, and energy.' Fill this room with these wonderful quality.

5. When your mind is focused on your breath, it cannot focus on another thing, person or distraction.

6. If you find yourself losing focus with distracting thoughts, bring your attention back to your breath.

7. Enjoy the moment for at least a few minutes and meditate longer as needed.

8. Smile and thank you for being in the present.

Guided Meditation with Props

Mantra

A mantra is a personal phrase, keywords, or scripture repeated several time in silence or in a soft whisper. Focusing on the mantra and its meaning will help quiet the mind. The repetition of the mantra can help reduce stress, calm the heart, and lower blood pressure. The practice of mantra keeps the mind steady and still.

Mudra

Mudras are hand gestures used during meditation to represent the unspoken language of blessings. Our fingers and thumb have the characteristics of the five natural elements (air, fire, water, earth, and space/ether) of life, which each serves a special function within the body. For example, Prayer Pose Mudra is represented by pressing the palms together in the center of your chest at your heart to neutralize the positive and negative energy of the mind.

Music

Music therapy during meditation has shown to increase relaxation, increase mental concentration, and help with anxiety disorders. Meditating with natural nature sound (i.e. sitting under a tree and listening to the wind blowing on the leaves) allows fresh oxygen to enter into the mind.

Aromatherapy

The use of essential oils can help ground and uplift your spirit during meditation. Essential oils can help bring micro particles to the brain which can increase focus and improve long-term memory.

Chakras System

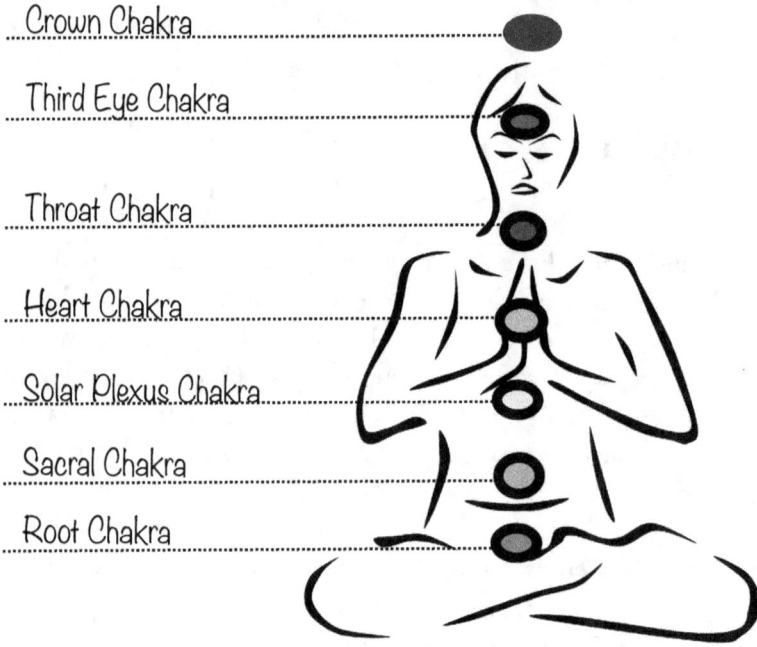

Crown Chakra

Third Eye Chakra

Throat Chakra

Heart Chakra

Solar Plexus Chakra

Sacral Chakra

Root Chakra

Chakras are the subtle energy centers in our body, where energy flows through in and throughout us. There are seven core chakras which can awaken or remain inactive based on our physical, emotional, and spiritual state. Yoga practice helps to balance the chakras and reveal area(s) that needs attention.

MY NOTES

MY NOTES

MY NOTES

MY NOTES

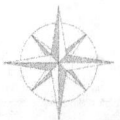

Vision Page for
Spiritual Wellness

MONTH:

Wellness	
WEEK # 1	**SMARTER Weekly Goals**
SUN	
MON	
TUES	
WED	
THURS	
FRI	
SAT	

Week # 1
Reflective Responses:

List ways you find peace in the midst of chaos. Learn to center your mind and uncover new lessons learned during these challenging time. Recite a mantra, use a mudra for guidance, listen to calming music, or meditate in silence.

_____

_____

_____

_____

_____

_____

_____

_____

_____

_____

_____

_____

_____

_____

_____

_____

_____

_____

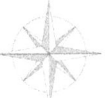 **Spiritual Wellness**

MONTH:

Wellness	
WEEK # 2	**SMARTER Weekly Goals**
SUN	
MON	
TUES	
WED	
THURS	
FRI	
SAT	

Week # 2
Reflective Responses:

List ways you can share respectfully your spiritual sacred space to offer peace, happiness, or joy to others. Are there ways you can learn to appreciate other types of spiritual wellness?

_____

_____

_____

_____

_____

_____

_____

_____

_____

_____

_____

_____

_____

_____

_____

_____

_____

_____

_____

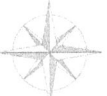 **Spiritual Wellness**

MONTH:

Wellness	
WEEK # 3	**SMARTER Weekly Goals**
SUN	
MON	
TUES	
WED	
THURS	
FRI	
SAT	

Week # 3
Reflective Responses:
Creative visualization is a technique that uses mental imagery to project the life you want. Where do you see yourself in 5 years? What impact do you want to make in the world? Can you make a SMARTER goal or one step forward today to move toward this vision?

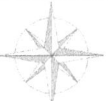 **Spiritual Wellness**

MONTH:

Wellness	
WEEK # 4	**SMARTER Weekly Goals**
SUN	
MON	
TUES	
WED	
THURS	
FRI	
SAT	

Week # 4
Reflective Responses:

List the people who have shaped your personality in the different stages of your life (childhood, adolescence, teenage years, etc …). Now, ask yourself: what impressions are you making on others?

_____

_____

_____

_____

_____

_____

_____

_____

_____

_____

_____

_____

_____

_____

_____

_____

_____

_____

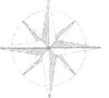 **Spiritual Wellness**

MONTH:

Wellness	
WEEK # 5	**SMARTER Weekly Goals**
SUN	
MON	
TUES	
WED	
THURS	
FRI	
SAT	

Week # 5
Reflective Responses:

List the things that you would like to see done for your local community. Are there ways you can contribute to this vision of a greater community? What public service can you engage in (i.e. volunteer, participate in town hall meeting or create your own social change etc…)?

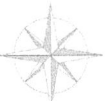 **Spiritual Wellness**

MONTH:

Wellness	
WEEK # 6	**SMARTER Weekly Goals**
SUN	
MON	
TUES	
WED	
THURS	
FRI	
SAT	

Week # 6
Reflective Responses:

List your favorite quotes that make feel inspired. What
can you do in the next five minutes to make this call to
action into a reality?

_____

_____

_____

_____

_____

_____

_____

_____

_____

_____

_____

_____

_____

_____

_____

_____

_____

_____

_____

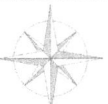 **Spiritual Wellness**

MONTH:

Wellness	
WEEK # 7	**SMARTER Weekly Goals**
SUN	
MON	
TUES	
WED	
THURS	
FRI	
SAT	

Week # 7
Reflective Responses:

List your favorite places to relax. Describe these places in term of the five senses (relaxation that eases the sight, sound, taste, touch, and scent). Can you use creative visualization to project and recreate these details in your current environment?

_____

_____

_____

_____

_____

_____

_____

_____

_____

_____

_____

_____

_____

_____

_____

_____

_____

_____

_____

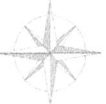 **Spiritual Wellness**

WELLNESS REFLECTIONS:

What brought you positive energy from this dimension of wellness? What were your hopes, inspirations, and dreams during this new change?

What brought you negative energy from this dimension of wellness? Did you experience any obstacles, distractions, or guilty feeling toward new change?

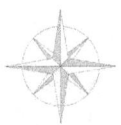

Social Wellness

Social wellness is how well we relate to our friends and family. We must learn to be open minded and to communicate openly with empathy. When you try to aim for perfection or to be *always* right, you learn the opportunity to hear the other person's perspective. It then becomes difficult to connect with others whole-heartedly. When we fail to listen with our hearts, communication becomes one-way, a monolog rather than a dialogue. Even though we may have different communication styles, we all possess a heart that can listen and accept unconditionally.

According to Gary Chapman, an author and researcher, to be effective listeners, we need to be aware of the five different communication styles:

- Sharing Gifts
- Providing Services
- Saying Words
- Spending Quality Time
- Giving Personal Touch

There are many different types of personality traits assessments, tests, and tools available. We behave and react based on our preferences, values, culture, genetics and non-genetic influences. Try one of the tools that is either based on western philosophy or eastern-philosophy (see the following tables)

Western Philosophy-Based Personality Assessment

Types	Description
Eysenck's personality Inventory (EPI)	Personality differences are based on genetic inheritance and the test measures temperament in terms of three qualities: 1) Extraversion, 2) Neuroticism, 3) Socialization
Holland Codes	Careers choice based upon personality types: Realistic (Doers), Investigative (Thinkers), Artistic (Creators), Social (Helpers), Enterprising (Persuaders), and Conventional (Organizers)
Myers–Briggs Type Indicator (MBTI)	How people perceive the world and make decisions based on personality types and cognitive functions: 1) Extraversion/Introversion, 2) Sensing/Intuition, 3) Thinking/Feeling, 4) Judging/Perceiving
DISC assessment	Focuses on four different behavioral traits: Dominance, inducement, submission, and compliance.
Big Five personality traits	Five factors have been defined as openness to experience, conscientiousness, extraversion, agreeableness, and neuroticism, often listed under the acronyms OCEAN
Pearson-Marr Archetype Indicator (PMAI)	Seek to become aware of 12 different archetypes in humans: Innocent, Orphan, Warrior, Caregiver, Seeker, Lover, Destroyer, Creator, Ruler, Magician, Sage, and Jester

Eastern Philosophy-Based Personality Assessment

Types	Description
Enneagram of Personality,	Balance the nine types along with their basic relationships : Reformer, Helper, Motivator, Romantic, Thinker, Skeptic, Enthusiast, Leader, Peacemaker.
Ayurveda and Body Types	Balance the three body types (doshas) with the different seasons for diet and lifestyle: Vata, Pitta, and Kapha
Five Chinese Elements	Five archetypal personalities associated with each element: "Pioneer" for Wood, "Wizard" for Fire, "Peacemaker" for Earth, "Alchemist" for Metal, and "Philosopher" for Water.
Yin/Yang	How opposite energy is balanced to maintain harmony. Yin represents the feminine calming quality, where as Yang represents the masculine power and strength.
Chinese Zodiac Horoscopes	Personality traits are represented by 12 animals that rules the year of your birth: Tiger, Sheep, Dog, Horse, Rabbit, Monkey, Pig, Dragon, Rat, Rooster, Snake, and Ox.
Seven Chakra Energy Bodies	In Hindu traditions, each person possess seven energy bodies (chakra) that impacts mood, energy, and life choices:
12 Zodiacal Signs	Personality types are based on astrological events on your birth date: Aries, Taurus, Gemini, Cancer, Leo, Virgo, Libra, Scorpio, Sagittarius, Capricorn, Aquarius, and Pisces.

Take one (or more) of the personality assessments/tests. Jot down your findings. Do you agree or disagree with these results? Did the findings surprise you? (and why or why not?)

MY NOTES

MY NOTES

MY NOTES

MY NOTES

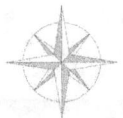

Vision Page for
Social Wellness

MONTH:

Wellness	
WEEK # 1	**SMARTER Weekly Goals**
SUN	
MON	
TUES	
WED	
THURS	
FRI	
SAT	

Week # 1
Reflective Responses:

Be an active listener and observer. During a conversation, resist the temptation to think and plan what to say next. Instead, focus on the tone and how the words are spoken by the other person. Describe how this made you and the other person feel.

_____

_____

_____

_____

_____

_____

_____

_____

_____

_____

_____

_____

_____

_____

_____

_____

_____

_____

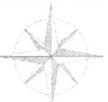 **Social Wellness**

MONTH:

Wellness	
WEEK # 2	**SMARTER Weekly Goals**
SUN	
MON	
TUES	
WED	
THURS	
FRI	
SAT	

Week # 2
Reflective Responses:

Test your vibes. When you walk into a room, bring your biggest sunshine with you and talk with your heart and not with your mind. How did your body feel afterward? How was your interaction with others?

_____

_____

_____

_____

_____

_____

_____

_____

_____

_____

_____

_____

_____

_____

_____

_____

_____

_____

_____

MONTH:

Wellness	
WEEK # 3	**SMARTER Weekly Goals**
SUN	
MON	
TUES	
WED	
THURS	
FRI	
SAT	

Week # 3
Reflective Responses:

Describe your social network: your closest friends, mentors, and acquaintances. Our personality is molded by genetics and external influencers. Do you see any differences in the personality traits in your current network of friends compared to the network of friends you had ten years ago? Why?

_____

_____

_____

_____

_____

_____

_____

_____

_____

_____

_____

_____

_____

_____

_____

_____

_____

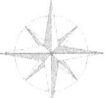 **Social Wellness**

MONTH:

Wellness	
WEEK # 4	**SMARTER Weekly Goals**
SUN	
MON	
TUES	
WED	
THURS	
FRI	
SAT	

Week # 4
Reflective Responses:

List your ideal friend or partner. Why? Do you see these characteristics in yourself? Did you see any of these traits change from years to years?

_____

_____

_____

_____

_____

_____

_____

_____

_____

_____

_____

_____

_____

_____

_____

_____

_____

_____

_____

_____

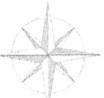 **Social Wellness**

MONTH:

Wellness	
WEEK # 5	**SMARTER Weekly Goals**
SUN	
MON	
TUES	
WED	
THURS	
FRI	
SAT	

Week # 5
Reflective Responses:

List the ways you approach a new stranger(s) at a party. What would you say? What is your 10-second elevator pitch?

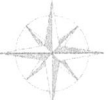

Social Wellness

MONTH:

Wellness	
WEEK # 6	**SMARTER Weekly Goals**
SUN	
MON	
TUES	
WED	
THURS	
FRI	
SAT	

Week # 6
Reflective Responses:

Is there any social drama in my life right? Are there any old grudges and unspoken tensions holding me back? What drama must I let go of?

_____

_____

_____

_____

_____

_____

_____

_____

_____

_____

_____

_____

_____

_____

_____

_____

_____

_____

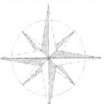 **Social Wellness**

MONTH:

Wellness	
WEEK # 7	**SMARTER Weekly Goals**
SUN	
MON	
TUES	
WED	
THURS	
FRI	
SAT	

Week # 7
Reflective Responses:

How are my deepest fears holding me back from evolving into a well-designed self? What has been my biggest barrier? Can I create a supportive community or environmental triggers to address this obstacle?

_____

_____

_____

_____

_____

_____

_____

_____

_____

_____

_____

_____

_____

_____

_____

_____

_____

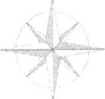 **Social Wellness**

WELLNESS REFLECTIONS:

What brought you positive energy from this dimension of wellness? What were your hopes, inspirations, and dreams during this new change?

What brought you negative energy from this dimension of wellness? Did you experience any obstacles, distractions, or guilty feeling toward new change?

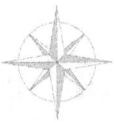

Occupational Wellness

Occupational wellness is how well we feel toward our purpose in the workplace. You could think of occupational wellness as work wellness or career wellness. Is your current career path meeting your needs, including your basic survival needs, such as income and job security, and fulfilling your dreams, your vision, and your mission in life?

A very healthy state of occupational wellness is a person who's doing exactly what they want to do in life and is comfortable and content with their personal and financial situation and plans.

But in our busy world, we tend to get distracted. Use these SMARTER work tips to concentrate your energy to be effective and efficient.

80/20 Rule: Assess your key assets that help you achieve more with less time and effort. Concentrate your time, resources and effort into 20% that will produce 80% of your maximal results, productivity and projected outcomes (i.e. losing weight, getting promotion … etc.).

Parkinson's Law: Work expands to fill the time and space available for it to be done. Thus, the more undefined time you give for the work, the more time it will take for the work to get done. Limit or restrict your time with a deadline. As the length of time for the task became shorter, the task becomes completed in the most cost-efficient and cost-effective way.

"50/30/20" Rule to Financial Health

When our money problems get out of control, the stress of finance can impact your health, all the dimensions of wellness, and your relationships with loved ones.

How much we want to work or need to work is closely knitted to the 7 dimensions of wellness. The old saying, "to live *within* your means", no longer applies to the current economy (as of 2017). Instead, the new rule of thumb is to "live *below* your means."

Although there is no magic number that will make you 100% in perfect financial health, there is a healthy range that can help you feel balanced, fulfilled and financially independent.

Developed by the economist Elizabeth Warren, here is a formula that is useful and easy to remember to balance your financial health.

Your take-home paycheck can be broken down as:

50% (or less) for NEEDS:
About half of your payment can be used to pay the "must haves" needed for basic survival such as food, rent/mortgage, basic clothing, and transportation.

30% (or less) for WANTS:
About less than a third of your payment can be used for your personal uses, entertainment, fun activities (yoga class, movie, and outing), traveling, and shopping. Reward yourself for a job well done living below your means.

20% (or more) for SAVINGS:
About 20% (or more) of your payment goes toward your savings and retirement funds. Aim to save up to 9 months of salary as an emergency fund.

MY NOTES

MY NOTES

MY NOTES

MY NOTES

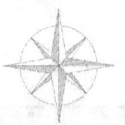

Vision Page for
Occupational Wellness

MONTH:

Wellness	
WEEK # 1	**SMARTER Weekly Goals**
SUN	
MON	
TUES	
WED	
THURS	
FRI	
SAT	

Week # 1
Reflective Responses:

What tasks do you spend 80% of the time doing that bring in 20% of the returns (i.e., checking email over and over, writing memos, taking a long time to make basic and unimportant decisions, etc.)? How can you change to use 20% of your time to yield 80% of your benefits?

_____

_____

_____

_____

_____

_____

_____

_____

_____

_____

_____

_____

_____

_____

_____

_____

_____

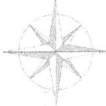 **Occupational Wellness**

MONTH:

Wellness	
WEEK # 2	**SMARTER Weekly Goals**
SUN	
MON	
TUES	
WED	
THURS	
FRI	
SAT	

Week # 2
Reflective Responses:

The 80/20 rule applies to other dimensions of wellness. What are the 20% of behaviors that cause 80% of the problems in your relationships? Can you and your partner focus on maximizing the 80% of joy and happiness in the relationships?

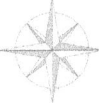 **Occupational Wellness**

MONTH:

Wellness	
WEEK # 3	**SMARTER Weekly Goals**
SUN	
MON	
TUES	
WED	
THURS	
FRI	
SAT	

Week # 3
Reflective Responses:

What is the 20% of your work that gets you 80% of the credit and recognition from your team or boss? With the remaining time, how can you use the recognition to further advance your current career, purpose and vision?

_____

_____

_____

_____

_____

_____

_____

_____

_____

_____

_____

_____

_____

_____

_____

_____

_____

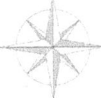 **Occupational Wellness**

MONTH:

Wellness	
WEEK # 4	**SMARTER Weekly Goals**
SUN	
MON	
TUES	
WED	
THURS	
FRI	
SAT	

Week # 4
Reflective Responses:

Become aware of how the work place affects your mood.
Do you notice how you feel after work? Does this feeling
linger its way to home? Describe the ways you can learn
to observe your mood and learn not to absorb any
negative energy from the workplace to your home life.

_____

_____

_____

_____

_____

_____

_____

_____

_____

_____

_____

_____

_____

_____

_____

_____

_____

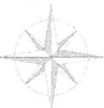 **Occupational Wellness**

MONTH:

Wellness	
WEEK # 5	**SMARTER Weekly Goals**
SUN	
MON	
TUES	
WED	
THURS	
FRI	
SAT	

Week # 5
Reflective Responses:

Be mindful of the energy in your living and work space. When you interact with a co-worker, study them. Listen to what and how they are saying. What personality traits do you see at your workplace? Can you learn to diffuse strong, negative energy to keep the peace?

_____

_____

_____

_____

_____

_____

_____

_____

_____

_____

_____

_____

_____

_____

_____

_____

_____

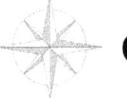 **Occupational Wellness**

MONTH:

WEEK # 6	SMARTER Weekly Goals
Wellness	
SUN	
MON	
TUES	
WED	
THURS	
FRI	
SAT	

Week # 6
Reflective Responses:

When you receive a work assignment, what is your process for managing time and resources to complete the task? If you were to apply the "Parkinson's Law" where work expands into the given space of time, how would you change your management style?

_____

_____

_____

_____

_____

_____

_____

_____

_____

_____

_____

_____

_____

_____

_____

_____

_____

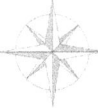 **Occupational Wellness**

MONTH:

Wellness	
WEEK # 7	**SMARTER Weekly Goals**
SUN	
MON	
TUES	
WED	
THURS	
FRI	
SAT	

Week # 7
Reflective Responses:

Let's make-believe. Pick one and reflect.

- ❑ If you were elected to be president, list the changes you'd like to see in the world.
- ❑ If you just won the lottery, list how you would spend the money.
- ❑ If you were an astronaut, list what you'd like to see in space.

_____

_____

_____

_____

_____

_____

_____

_____

_____

_____

_____

_____

_____

_____

_____

_____

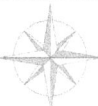 **Occupational Wellness**

WELLNESS REFLECTIONS:

What brought you positive energy from this dimension of wellness? What were your hopes, inspirations, and dreams during this new change?

What brought you negative energy from this dimension of wellness? Did you experience any obstacles, distractions, or guilty feeling toward new change?

#WellnessPlanDNA

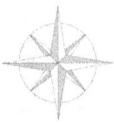

Environmental Wellness

Environmental wellness is being aware of our surroundings, assess our knowledge and understand what motivates us and demotivates us. Once we understand we need to have a change, we can than develop a self-management plan for ourselves and receive support among our community to keep us on track.

1. **Mini-incremental Change.** One push-up per day. One minute meditation. One flight of stairs at work. Park a block from your work place.

2. **Schedule Mini-breaks throughout the day.** With our smartphone technology, you can send a reminder to yourself to do your mini-habit (i.e. 10-minute crunches, 2-minute meditation, or 10-minute walk … etc.)

3. **Block off a 'Health Appointment' with yourself in your calendar.** We often feel guilty for taking the time to exercise when we feel we can use that time to work more, spend time with others, or make errands. The next time someone wants to use your time during your workout time, you can simply say 'you have a health appointment.'

4. **Remove distractors and add a booster to your surroundings.** If you want to make a habit of exercising regularly, place your running shoes and workout gear near the door, or bring them to work with you. Remove or minimize any possibility for distractors and delay in decision-making.

Change Your Environment.
Change Your Genes

The Power of Epigenetics

Environmental wellness has two sides: internal and external environment. The internal environmental wellness (your immune system, nervous system, digestion system, and muscular system) is impacted by the external environmental (the air you breathe, the nutrients in the food you eat, and the toxins around your surrounding).

The science of wellness tells us that environmental factors can impact the expression of our genes. What we eat, taste, feel, smell, and sense may seem to have a transient impact, but in reality, they may have a long-lasting effect. The lingering impact can" imprint" onto our DNA, through a process called "epigenetic mechanism." These factors (stress, toxins, immune factors, nutrients) can structurally change our DNA, by turning on or off our genes. The epigenetic mechanism can also limit the expression of important genes, increase the expression of bad genes, or decrease the quantity of gene products needed for proper functions (such as fighting against toxic exposure that can impact the growth of tumor cells). Epigenetics is a powerful gene modifier.

The microbiome is the bacterial community in your guts that helps you digest and process food in the stomach as well as the "food for thoughts" in your brain. Having a healthy gut bacteria is connected to a healthy development of cognition functions, effective immune system, and physical fitness.

MY NOTES

MY NOTES

MY NOTES

MY NOTES

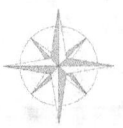

Vision Page for
Environmental Wellness

MONTH:

Wellness	
WEEK # 1	**SMARTER Weekly Goals**
SUN	
MON	
TUES	
WED	
THURS	
FRI	
SAT	

Week # 1
Reflective Responses:

List all of your favorite things about winter (food, things to do, watch, and travel). Does your diet, routine, or lifestyle change during this season? What mini-habit can you add to foster a healthy environment? Healthy gut makes a healthy brain.

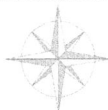 **Environmental Wellness**

MONTH:

Wellness	
WEEK # 2	**SMARTER Weekly Goals**
SUN	
MON	
TUES	
WED	
THURS	
FRI	
SAT	

Week # 2
Reflective Responses:

List all of your favorite things about summer (food, things to do, watch, and travel). Does your diet, routine, or lifestyle change during this season? What mini-habit can you add to foster a healthy environment? Healthy gut makes a healthy brain.

_____

_____

_____

_____

_____

_____

_____

_____

_____

_____

_____

_____

_____

_____

_____

_____

_____

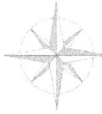 **Environmental Wellness**

MONTH:

Wellness	
WEEK # 3	**SMARTER Weekly Goals**
SUN	
MON	
TUES	
WED	
THURS	
FRI	
SAT	

Week # 3
Reflective Responses:

List all of your favorite things about autumn (food, things to do, watch, and travel). Does your diet, routine, or lifestyle change during this season? What mini-habit can you add to foster a healthy environment? Healthy gut makes a healthy brain.

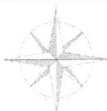 **Environmental Wellness**

MONTH:

Wellness	
WEEK # 4	**SMARTER Weekly Goals**
SUN	
MON	
TUES	
WED	
THURS	
FRI	
SAT	

Week # 4
Reflective Responses:

List all of your favorite things about spring (food, things to do, watch, and travel). Does your diet, routine, or lifestyle change during this season? What mini-habit can you add to foster a healthy environment? Healthy gut makes a healthy brain.

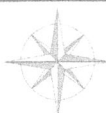 **Environmental Wellness**

MONTH:

Wellness	
WEEK # 5	**SMARTER Weekly Goals**
SUN	
MON	
TUES	
WED	
THURS	
FRI	
SAT	

Week # 5
Reflective Responses:

Keeping your body hydrated is important to optimize your physical and mental capacity. How many glasses of water do you drink (not including tea, coffee, or soft drink)? Drink a glass of warm water with lemon every morning for one week and then, reflect how your body and mind feel during this personal experiment.

_____

_____

_____

_____

_____

_____

_____

_____

_____

_____

_____

_____

_____

_____

_____

_____

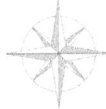 **Environmental Wellness**

MONTH:

Wellness	
WEEK # 6	**SMARTER Weekly Goals**
SUN	
MON	
TUES	
WED	
THURS	
FRI	
SAT	

Week # 6
Reflective Responses:

If you've been on a diet or weight management plan for some time, it is not unusual to feel a little fatigue from developing new habits. This is when 'self-defeating' thoughts sink into your mind. Watch out (don't go for that extra cookie). Reflect how you can fight the self-sabotaging behaviors.

_____

_____

_____

_____

_____

_____

_____

_____

_____

_____

_____

_____

_____

_____

_____

_____

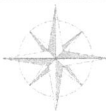 **Environmental Wellness**

MONTH:

Wellness	
WEEK # 7	**SMARTER Weekly Goals**
SUN	
MON	
TUES	
WED	
THURS	
FRI	
SAT	

Week # 7
Reflective Responses:

As you were making new changes, describes moments where you felt you had to use extraordinary willpower to control the urge to revert to old behaviors. Do you think you can remove environmental triggers to eliminate these temptations?

_____

_____

_____

_____

_____

_____

_____

_____

_____

_____

_____

_____

_____

_____

_____

_____

_____

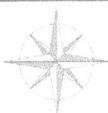 **Environmental Wellness**

WELLNESS REFLECTIONS:

What brought you positive energy from this dimension of wellness? What were your hopes, inspirations, and dreams during this new change?

What brought you negative energy from this dimension of wellness? Did you experience any obstacles, distractions, or guilty feeling toward new change?

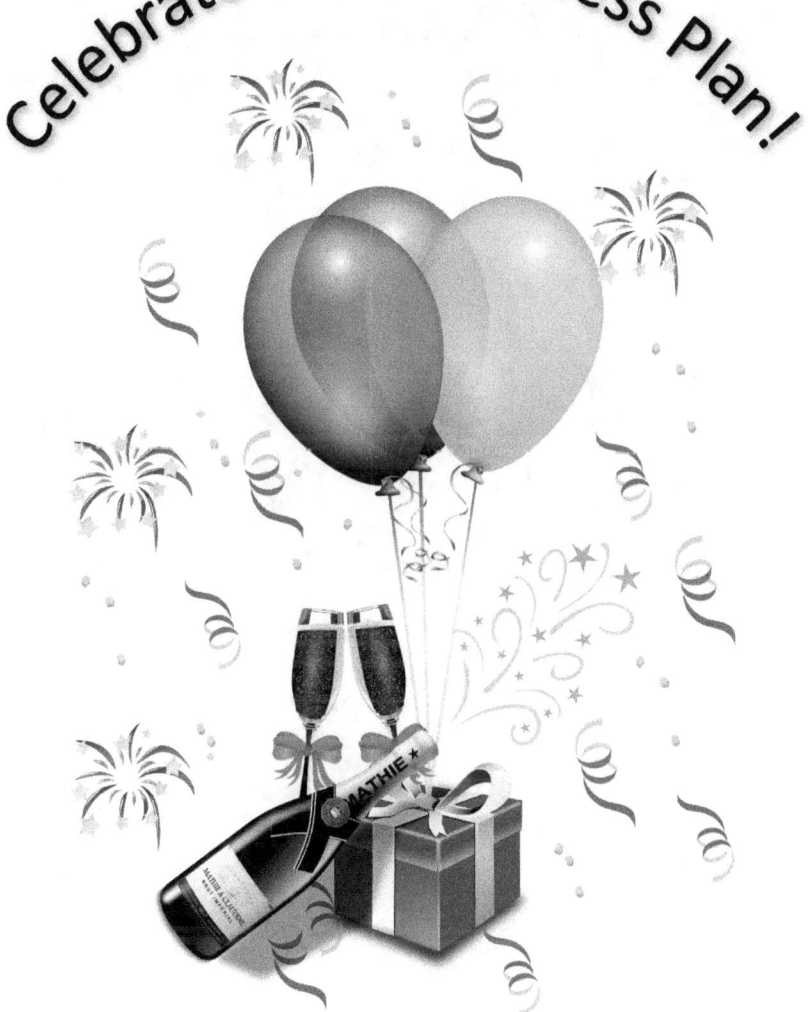

Celebrate Your Wellness Plan!

The Transformation I will see in myself now

(Describe or draw the newly well-designed you).

Dating the Well-Designed Me

To celebrate the new transformed you, treat yourself on a date with you! Here are some ideas:

- Read a love poem to yourself.

- Spend 15 minutes daydreaming looking at the clouds.

- Go to a shoe store and try out a new pair of fun shoes.

- Buy yourself a beautiful hand-held mirror to say "thank you YOU".

- Declutter your closer at once a month to open space in your heart and mind. Buy yourself a new outfit.

- Send a surprise postcard to yourself and what you saw that day.

- Try a new workout class for fun this week (usually, studio offer a free first class)

- Write a letter to your younger self.

- Phone an old friend and talk (not texting).

- Enjoy a cup of coffee or tea at your café with a book.

- Walk around the neighborhood and get to know your local small business owners.

- Buy yourself a bunch of flowers/roses and a box of chocolates with a written card saying "thank you for caring for me!"

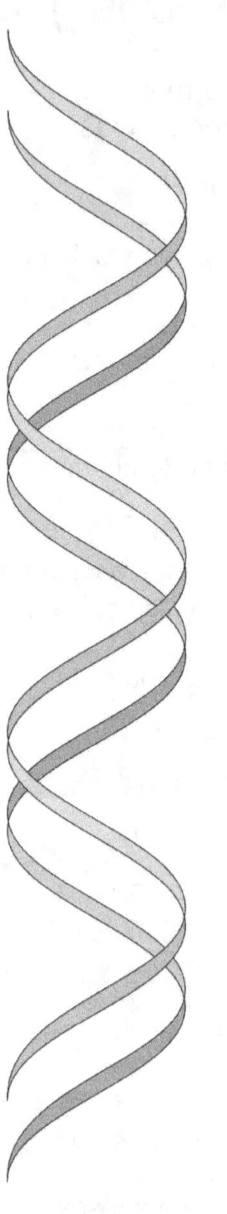

Part 4
References
&
Resources

References

Books

Chapman, Gary. *The 5 Love Languages: The Secret to Love that Lasts*. Chicago: Northfield Publishing. 2014.

Chopra, Deepak. *The Seven Spiritual Laws of Success: A Practical Guide to the Fulfillment of Your Dreams*. San Rafael: Amber-Allen Publishing. 2011.

Covey, Stephen. *The 7 Habits of Highly Effective People: Powerful Lessons in Personal Change*. New York: RosettaBooks. 2011

Duhigg, Charles. *The Power of Habit: Why We Do What We Do in Life and Business*. New York: Random House. 2012.

Goleman, Daniel. *Emotional Intelligence: Why It Can Matter More Than IQ*. New York: Bantam. 2011.

Godwin, M. *Who Are You? 101 Ways Of Seeing Yourself - From Archetypes And Chakras To Enneagrams And Sun Signs*., an identity-kit of physical, spiritual, mental and emotional self-test. New York: Penguin / Compass. 2000.

Kahneman, Daniel. *Thinking, Fast and Slow*. New York: Farra, Straus, and Giroux. 2011.

McGonigal, Kelly. *The Willpower Instinct: How Self-Control Works, Why It Matters, and What You Can Do to Get More of It*. New York: Avery. 2011.

Pollan, Michael. *In Defense of Food*. New York: Penguin Book. 2009.

Press, Zenergy. The SMARTER Method Planner Journal.

Reynolds, Gretchen. *The First 20 Minutes: Surprising Science Reveals How We Can Exercise Smarter, Live Longer.* New York: Avery. 2012.

Rock, David. *Your Brain at Work.* New York: HarperCollins. 2009 .

Stanley, Thomas and Danko, William. *The Millionaire Next Door.* New York: RosettaBooks. 2010.

Orman, Suze. *The 9 Steps to Financial Freedom: Practical and Spiritual Steps So You Can Stop Worrying.* New York: Crown Business. 1999.

Stauth, Cameron and Singh Khalsa D. *Meditation As Medicine: Activate the Power of Your Natural Healing Force.* New York: Atria Books. 2011.

Williamson, Marianne. *A Return to Love: Reflections on the Principles of A Course in Miracles.* San Francisco: HarperOne. 2009.

Websites:
National Institute of Complementary and Integrative Medicine https://nccih.nih.gov

HeartMath Institute https://www.heartmath.org

ZenOmix Institute of Health and Wellness www.zenomixinstitute.com

Resources

About ZenOmix Institute
of Health and Wellness

ZenOmix Institute of Health and Wellness is a unique wellness space which provides life-long learners with a variety of inspiration to manage their overall health, inner beauty, and wellness. We offer science-based approaches to healthy living and aging.

Make the positive lifestyle change you've been wanting; see what ZenOmix Institute has to offer you. Here, you will become a part of a caring community toward personalized healing through our well-designed words and actions.

- Publications (books, newsletter, social blog)

- Monthly private membership program

- Online courses on health, fitness and wellness

- Yoga, Pilates, and Barre classes

Sign up to become a member at ZenOmix Institute and receive free resources, videos and audiobooks.

www.zenomixinstitute.com

email: info@zenomixinstitute.com

Join the Mindful Movement

www.zenomixinstitute.com

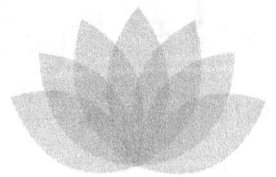

www.ingramcontent.com/pod-product-compliance
Lightning Source LLC
Chambersburg PA
CBHW072043280526
45788CB00006B/2159